ELEGANT TRANSFORMATION: INTERMITTENT FASTING FOR WOMEN OVER 5O

THE EASIEST WAY TO LOOSE WEIGHT, BOOST YOUR ENERGY AND OVERCOME AGEING SPELLS

BY

Kathryn J. Woodberry

DISCLAIMER

It is very important to speak with a trained healthcare provider before beginning any new eating plan, notably intermittent fasting, especially if you're a woman over 50. Although there are many health advantages to intermittent fasting, such as better metabolic health and weight control, it might not be the right choice for everyone.

Women over 50 may react differently to intermittent fasting due to certain health issues, including changes in hormones, altered metabolic rates, and possible dietary deficits. Therefore, before beginning an intermittent fasting regimen, it's essential to have a thorough health evaluation performed and to talk with a healthcare expert about your specific health objectives.

However, it's important to approach intermittent fasting carefully and customize it to suit each person's tastes, lifestyle, and medical background. It's critical to pay attention to your body, keep an eye out for any negative consequences, and modify the fasting schedule as necessary. If you develop extreme pain, dizziness, exhaustion, or any other worrisome symptoms, stop fasting and consult a physician.

This book you are about to explore right now is not intended to replace individual medical advice; rather, it acts as a general guide. Since every person's health situation is different, seeking expert advice is essential to determining if intermittent fasting is safe and appropriate for women over 50.

TABLE OF CONTENTS

ABOUT THE AUTHOR

Kathryn J. Woodberry is the author of Elegant Transformation: Intermittent Fasting for Women Over 50, The easiest way to lose weight, boost your energy and overcome aging spells.

Renowned nutritionist and wellness specialist Kathryn J. Woodberry has more than 20 years of expertise in the industry. Her work reflects her love for assisting people in achieving maximum health and vitality. She possesses postgraduate degrees in dietetics and nutrition.

In the field of intermittent fasting, especially for women over 50, Kathryn J. Woodberry has established herself as a reliable author thanks to her emphasis on evidence-based research and thorough knowledge of women's health concerns. She wants to encourage women to take charge of their health and age gracefully and vibrantly via her work.

Apart from being a writer, Kathryn J. Woodberry is also in high demand as a lecturer and educator, renowned for her captivating and educational talks on wellness, nutrition, and ageing well. She is committed to motivating people to make great life changes by imparting her knowledge and experience to them.

Women over 50 continue to benefit greatly from Kathryn J. Woodberry's caring approach and dedication to holistic health, which gives them the clarity and confidence to pursue their wellness and health objectives.

BOOK REVIEW

Elegant Transformation: Intermittent Fasting for Women Over 50 is a must-read for mature women looking to optimise their health and well-being through intermittent fasting.

Kathryn J. Woodberry provides a comprehensive and tailored approach to fasting that specifically addresses the unique needs and concerns of women.

This book emphasises safety and effectiveness. Recognizing that women over 50 may have different hormonal profiles and metabolic challenges, the author offers practical advice by addressing common concerns such as menopause, hormone fluctuations, and bone health, readers can feel confident in implementing fasting as part of their wellness routine because the book goes beyond weight loss to explore the essential benefits of intermittent fasting for women over 50. From improved cognitive function and mood to reduced inflammation and risk of chronic disease, the author highlights the potential for fasting to enhance overall health and quality of life. What sets this book apart is its holistic approach to ageing rather than viewing intermittent fasting as a standalone intervention, the author encourages readers to complement their fasting regimen with other healthy habits, such as regular exercise, stress management, and adequate sleep. This comprehensive approach fosters a synergistic effect, maximising the benefits of fasting while promoting long-term health and vitality. Also, the book is filled with practical tips, meal plans, and recipes tailored to the nutritional needs of women over 50. Whether you're new to intermittent fasting or a seasoned practitioner, you'll find valuable insights and actionable strategies to support your journey to healthier aging.

Elegant Transformation: Intermittent Fasting for Women Over 50 is a well-researched and also empowering resource that equips readers with the knowledge and tools they need to embrace intermittent fasting as a key component of their health and wellness routine. This book is sure to inspire and empower women over 50 to thrive as they age.

INTRODUCTION

Do you need help keeping your weight under control and your health intact without sacrificing flavour?

If so, you ought to pick up this book! After 50, your body undergoes major changes, making it more difficult to maintain or reduce weight. These changes are usually more pronounced in women, however they are sometimes seen in men. There will be a lot of changes that you'll notice, especially with your hormones as they slow down your metabolism and diminish your energy levels. How can you address these problems to improve your health and reduce your weight?

The answer is INTERMITTENT FASTING.

This book focuses specifically on methods that any woman over 50 may apply to age gracefully on her body while also managing her weight loss.

Women over 50 are increasingly adopting intermittent fasting as a way to maintain their health and control their weight. Numerous advantages can result from it, including greater energy, less inflammation, enhanced mental clarity, and improved general health.

Everything you need to know about intermittent fasting is covered in this book, including its advantages, techniques, and beneficial outcomes.

It is a useful tool for some over-50 women who have struggled with their weight for years and are now reaching their weight-loss objectives.

Fasting intermittently is a tactic rather than a diet, therefore you may decide the meals you want to eat, how long to adapt it for, and how the macronutrients are distributed. The durability of the diet may be improved by these factors as they tailor the fasting schedule to your dietary requirements, lifestyle, and favorite meals that will provide you with more satisfaction.

CHAPTER ONE

UNDERSTANDING INTERMITTENT FASTING

Intermittent fasting (IF) alternate between times when you eat and when you fast. It places more emphasis on when to eat foods than on what to eat. It also entails alternating between eating and fasting intervals. The body starts burning fat for energy during fasting periods as a result of depleting its stores of glycogen, or stored glucose which can lead to weight loss. Fasting also causes hormone levels to fluctuate and initiate a variety of cellular repair processes, all of which have a positive impact on health.

CATEGORIES OF INTERMITTENT FASTING

Intermittent fasting has categories therefore I will be suggesting you choose the category that best suits you and patiently wait for the excellent results, below are the categories of intermittent fasting.

• **Time-Restricted Eating:** This approach entails eating all of your meals during a predetermined window of time and fasting for a predetermined number of hours each day, usually between 12 and 20.

• **Alternate-Day Fasting:** This method alternates regular eating days with fasting days. Calorie consumption is drastically reduced or avoided during fasting days.

• **5:2 Diet:** This plan calls for eating regularly five days a week and substantially cutting calories (to 500–600) on the two non-consecutive days that you don't eat.

HEALTH BENEFITS

It might interest you to know that intermittent fasting has loads of benefits for aging. Ones especially for women over 50, here I will be listing some of the health benefits.

1.   **Weight reduction:** Intermittent fasting is a useful weight reduction strategy since it can result in calorie restriction and fat loss.

2.   **Enhanced Insulin Sensitivity:** Insulin sensitivity is enhanced by fasting, which may lower the risk of type 2 diabetes by regulating blood sugar levels.

3.   **Cellular Repair:** Autophagy, a mechanism that causes cells to eliminate damaged parts, is triggered by fasting and results in cellular regeneration and repair.

4.   **Brain Health:** Research indicates that fasting intermittently may enhance mental acuity, guard against neurodegenerative illnesses, and enhance cognitive function.

WHO CAN BENEFIT

Even while many people find that intermittent fasting is helpful, it's important to take individual aspects like age, gender, health, and lifestyle into account. Before beginning an intermittent fast, see a doctor, especially if you use medication or have underlying medical issues.

The first step to maximising intermittent fasting's potential health advantages is comprehending its guiding principles. You may maximise your health and well-being by thoughtfully and under appropriate supervision implementing intermittent fasting into your lifestyle.

<u>HOW DOES INTERMITTENT FASTING WORK?</u>

The way intermittent fasting operates is by alternating between eating and fasting intervals. Your body burns fat that has been stored as fuel throughout the fasting phase since there is no food coming in. Numerous health advantages may result from this, such as enhanced insulin sensitivity, weight loss, and cellular repair mechanisms. The two most popular fasting regimens are the 16/8 technique, which calls for 16 hours of fasting followed by an 8-hour window for eating, and the 5:2 approach, which calls for 5 days of regular eating followed by 2 days of drastically reduced calorie consumption.

BENEFITS OF INTERMITTENT FASTING FOR WOMEN OVER 50

By lowering calorie consumption and enhancing metabolic health, intermittent fasting provides weight control, which may aid in weight loss or management. Additionally, it improves insulin sensitivity, which is especially advantageous for women over 50 who may be more susceptible to type 2 diabetes and insulin resistance. According to some study, cardiovascular health parameters including blood pressure, cholesterol, and inflammatory markers are all improved by intermittent fasting. Intermittent fasting may promote brain health and lower the risk of age-related cognitive decline, according to new research. Autophagy, a cellular repair mechanism that eliminates damaged cells and may offer protection against age-related illnesses, is triggered by fasting. Additionally, it aids in the regulation of hormone levels such as ghrelin, insulin, and leptin, which can support the general health and hormonal balance of women over 50.

CHAPTER TWO

GETTING STARTED WITH INTERMITTENT FASTING

Naturally, the fact that intermittent fasting alternates between eating and fasting times makes this a fascinating feature of the practice.

I advise you to start by selecting a fasting plan from the Common techniques, such as the 16/8 method, which entails a 16-hour fast followed by an 8-hour window for eating. Additionally, there is the alternate day fasting approach, which entails fasting every other day, or the 5:2 method, which calls for eating regularly for 5 days while limiting calories to 500–600 on the other 2 non-consecutive days.

You must ease yourself into fasting as not everyone is experienced with it. This will help you feel more secure as you attempt to get back in shape. If you have never fasted before, begin by progressively extending the length of your fasts. Continually During times of fasting, be sure to keep hydrated by drinking lots of water, herbal tea, or black coffee to satisfy your appetite. To fuel your body, ensure you take meals like fruits, vegetables, lean proteins, and healthy fats during mealtime periods and concentrate on nutrient-dense foods.

Always pay attention to your body's signals of hunger and modify your fasting schedule accordingly. If you experience extreme exhaustion or illness, you should think about changing your strategy or seeing a medical expert.

Be patient with yourself and give yourself time to achieve great benefits. Your body may need some time to adjust to intermittent fasting, so don't anticipate a dramatic improvement right away.

ASSESSING YOUR HEALTH AND GOALS

Before beginning intermittent fasting, it's important to evaluate your goals and state of health. Ensure you seek advice from a physician or trained dietitian before beginning any new diet or fasting program, particularly if you have any underlying medical ailments or concerns. Identify your objectives, know exactly what you want, for instance you are trying to reach any other health-related goals, such as weight loss, better metabolic health, or more energy? Setting clear objectives for yourself will enable you to adjust your intermittent fasting strategy appropriately.

Evaluate your current health status to ascertain whether intermittent fasting is a good choice for you, take into account variables like your present weight, body composition, blood sugar, cholesterol, and general health.

Consider your lifestyle when selecting an intermittent fasting technique, consider your daily schedule, job obligations, fitness regimen, and social activities. Choose a fasting plan that suits your tastes and way of life.

Monitor changes in weight, body measurements, energy, mood, and general well-being to keep tabs on your progress over time. To make sure your fasting regimen is successful and sustainable for you, make any necessary adjustments.

Listen to your body, observe how intermittent fasting affects your body and note how it reacts. Should you have extreme hunger, exhaustion, lightheadedness, or any other negative consequences, you might want to adjust your strategy or consult a medical practitioner. You may create a safe, efficient, and long-lasting intermittent fasting plan for yourself by evaluating your goals and current health.

CHOOSING THE RIGHT INTERMITTENT FASTING PLAN

As previously said, there are several kinds of intermittent fasting regimens; the secret is to figure out which one best fits your needs, tastes, and health objectives. Here are a few well-liked choices to think about before making your decision:

1.   **16/8 METHOD:** This entails limiting meals to an 8-hour window and fasting for 16 hours every day. It is adaptable to most lifestyles and is rather simple to execute.

2.   **5:2 METHOD:** This strategy involves consuming 500–600 calories per day on two non-consecutive days while eating

regularly the other five days. Although it offers flexibility, on fasting days it demands more self control.

3.   **ALTERNATE DAY FASTING:** Switching back and forth between non-fasting and fasting days, during which you eat little to nothing. Although some people may find it difficult to follow this strategy consistently over the long run, it can be useful for losing weight.

4.   **EAT-STOP-EAT:** This entails fasting once or twice a week for a whole 24-hour period. Going a whole day without eating is easy, but for some people it might be challenging.

5.   **WARRIOR DIET:** This diet entails a single, substantial meal consumed within a 4-hour window and 20 hours of fasting every day. It might not be appropriate for everyone due to its intense nature.

<h1 align="center">CHAPTER THREE</h1>

<h1 align="center">THE SCIENCE BEHIND INTERMITTENT FASTING</h1>

Scientifically, it is possible to achieve health advantages through intermittent fasting (IF), which has garnered interest, so I have carefully and explained below the impact of science behind intermittent fasting.

WEIGHT REDUCTION

By lowering caloric intake and raising fat burning, IF can result in weight reduction. It may help target stubborn belly fat and be just as successful in losing weight as typical calorie restriction, according to studies.

BETTER INSULIN SENSITIVITY

IF can raise insulin sensitivity, which is important for controlling blood sugar levels and lowering the chance of type 2 diabetes. Additionally, it could enhance blood sugar regulation and decrease fasting insulin levels.

CELLULAR REPAIR AND AUTOPHAGY

Autophagy is the mechanism by which cells recycle damaged parts for energy and eliminate them from the body when fasting. This might aid in preventing illnesses including cancer and neurological conditions.

Some other discoveries are

DECREASED INFLAMMATION: Heart disease, cancer, and Alzheimer's are just a few of the illnesses that are associated with chronic inflammation. It has been demonstrated that IF lowers inflammatory indicators in the body, which may lessen the chance of developing several illnesses.

HEART HEALTH: By reducing blood pressure, triglycerides, cholesterol, and inflammatory indicators, intermittent fasting may enhance heart health. A decreased risk of heart disease and stroke is a result of these variables.

BRAIN HEALTH: According to some study, IF may help maintain brain health by encouraging the synthesis of BDNF, a protein involved in memory, learning, and cognitive function. It could help guard against cognitive deterioration brought on by aging.

IMPACT ON HORMONES AND METABOLISM

An improvement in insulin sensitivity, an increase in fat burning, and better management of hunger can result from intermittent fasting's beneficial effects on hormone levels and metabolism. Individual reactions to intermittent fasting (IF) may differ, therefore as previously said, it's critical to pay attention to your body's signals and modify your fasting regimen accordingly.

This is how IF impacts metabolism and hormones:

1. **Insulin:** IF can increase insulin sensitivity, which will result in less insulin during fasting intervals and enhanced blood sugar regulation. This helps lower the risk of type 2 diabetes and insulin resistance.

2. **Growth Hormone (GH):** GH levels rise during periods of fasting, especially prolonged fasts. Growth of muscles, fat metabolism, and general cellular repair are all impacted by growth hormone (GH).

3. **Noradrenaline (norepinephrine):** Increasing noradrenaline levels during a fast might speed up metabolism and encourage fat burning. This facilitates the release of stored energy for usage during fasting.

4. **Cortisol:** Although cortisol levels can increase during fasting, they usually drop back to normal after consistent fasting. It is critical to control stress levels and get enough sleep since long-term increase of cortisol can have detrimental consequences on metabolism and general health.

5. **Leptin:** Also referred to as the "satiety hormone," leptin controls appetite and the distribution of calories. Increased leptin sensitivity has been linked to IF in some studies, which may aid in appetite management and weight loss.

6. **Ghrelin:** Often referred to as the "hunger hormone," ghrelin rises when the stomach is empty and falls when food is consumed. Fasting can raise ghrelin levels momentarily, but over time, they usually level out, resulting in less hunger and better control over appetite.

7. **Thyroid Hormones:** A brief fast may momentarily lower thyroid hormone levels, according to some study. That being said, this is often a natural reaction to store energy during a fast and does not always signify thyroid problems.

EFFECTS ON AGEING AND LONGEVITY

The information that is now available indicates that intermittent fasting (IF) may have advantages for encouraging long life and good ageing, even if the field of study on IF and ageing is still developing. IF must, however, be incorporated into a well-rounded lifestyle that consists of frequent exercise, a diet high in nutrients, and other healthful practices.

Research has examined the possible impacts of intermittent fasting (IF) on aging and lifespan, and it has identified many pathways by which IF might have these effects.

1. **Cellular Repair and Autophagy:** Autophagy is the mechanism by which cells recycle damaged parts for energy and eliminate them from the body when fasting. This process of clearing out damaged molecules and malfunctioning organelles from the cell may help prevent age-related decline and increase lifespan.

2. **Decreased Inflammation:** Aging and age-related illnesses are linked to chronic inflammation. It has been demonstrated that IF lowers inflammatory indicators in the body, which may help prevent age-related illnesses including cancer, heart disease, and neurological disorders as well as slow down the aging process.

3. **Better Metabolic Health:** By lowering insulin resistance, enhancing blood sugar regulation, and encouraging fat reduction, IF can enhance metabolic health. These metabolic enhancements may lead to a longer, healthier life expectancy and are linked to a decreased risk of age-related disorders.

4. **Increased Production of Neuroprotective Factors:** Research indicates that IF may boost the generation of neuroprotective factors, such as brain-derived neurotrophic factor (BDNF) and other factors that support brain health and may help fend off neurodegenerative illnesses like Alzheimer's and age-related cognitive decline.

5. **Enhanced Stress Resistance:** The body experiences mild stress during fasting, which sets off adaptive reactions that strengthen the body's defenses against stress and encourage cellular resilience. These changes may lengthen life expectancy by providing protection against aging-related harm.

MANAGING MENOPAUSE SYMPTOMS WITH INTERMITTENT FASTING

There are several packages (symptoms) associated with menopause, so it's critical to be aware of them. You should also be aware that, while individual reactions may differ, intermittent fasting may be able to assist manage these symptoms. Here are some possible effects of IF on particular menopausal symptoms

1. **WEIGHT CONTROL:** Hormonal changes and slowing metabolism during menopause cause many women to gain

weight. By encouraging fat reduction and enhancing metabolic health, IF might help control weight and perhaps avoid or lessen weight gain during this period.

2. **NIGHT SWEATS AND HOT FLASHES:** Although there isn't much data focused on IF and hot flashes, several women have found that when they follow an IF program, their night sweats and hot flashes go away.

3. **VIBRANT MOODS AND INTOLERANCE:** Improved insulin sensitivity and stable blood sugar levels brought on by IF may lessen agitation and assist regulate mood in women going through menopause by stabilizing hormone levels.

4. **CHANGES IN COGNITION AND BRAIN FOG:** According to some research, IF may improve neurogenesis and neurodegenerative processes in the brain, which in turn may help maintain brain health and cognitive performance. Menopause-related cognitive abnormalities and fogginess may be lessened by doing this.

5. **BONE HEALTH:** During menopause, preserving bone health requires eating a diet high in calcium and vitamin D. Although IF by itself has no direct effect on bone health, it is crucial for women who follow IF to make sure they are getting enough calcium and vitamin D in their diets to maintain bone health.

6. **DISTURBANCES IN SLEEP:** For some people, improved metabolic health and decreased inflammation brought on by IF may have a good impact on sleep quality. To maximize sleep during menopause, it's crucial to have a regular sleep pattern and adopt healthy sleeping practices.

CHAPTER FOUR

PRACTICAL TIPS FOR IMPLEMENTING INTERMITTENT FASTING

Planning and persistence are all you need to properly use intermittent fasting (IF). To begin, think about the following:

- **Gradually extending the length of your fasting periods:** As said previously in this book, if you're new to fasting, start out slowly. When you feel more at ease, progressively increase the duration of your overnight fast to 14, 16, or more hours. Begin with a 12-hour window

- **Selecting the appropriate approach:** Choose an IF technique that fits your tastes and way of living. Try out several fasting regimens, including the 16/8 technique, 5:2 method, or alternate-day fasting, to see which one suits you the best.

- **Remaining hydrated:** To keep hydrated and reduce hunger during fasting times, drink lots of water, herbal tea, or black coffee. Steer clear of calorically-rich or sugar-filled beverages since they may disrupt your fast.

- **Emphasizing nutrient-dense foods:** To promote general health and fuel your body, give entire foods like fruits, vegetables, lean meats, and healthy fats priority during meal periods. The advantages of fasting may be defeated if you overindulge in processed or high-calorie items during eating periods.

- **Listening to your body:** Pay attention to your body's signals of hunger and modify your fasting plan as necessary. If you experience extreme exhaustion, lightheadedness, or illness, you should think about changing your strategy or stopping the fast.

- **Meal planning:** Schedule your meals and snacks in advance to guarantee that you have wholesome selections accessible when you eat. This might lessen the likelihood of impulsive eating or grabbing for bad foods when you're hungry.

- **Being adaptable:** Life occurs, and there may be times when you don't feel like fasting or it's not practical for you. It's OK to be adaptable with your fasting schedule and make necessary adjustments in accordance with your situation and physical condition.

• **Remaining consistent:** Seeing benefits from intermittent fasting requires consistency. To get the most out of your selected fasting schedule, try to keep to it as much as possible, including on weekends and holidays.

• **Tracking your progress:** During your intermittent fasting regimen, note how you feel emotionally, psychologically, and physically. To determine the effect of IF on your health, track changes in your weight, body composition, energy levels, mood, and general well-being.

• **Looking for support:** You can get accountability, inspiration, and support for your IF journey by connecting with like-minded people online or by locating a fasting companion. You may overcome obstacles and maintain focus by talking to people about your experiences and advice.

<u>ADJUSTING INTERMITTENT FASTING FOR WOMEN OVER <u>50</u></u>

Women over 50 can modify their intermittent fasting by taking their hormonal fluctuations, metabolism, and dietary requirements into account. For women over fifty, modifying intermittent fasting entails taking individual requirements into consideration and modifying as needed to promote health and wellbeing throughout this phase of life. Here are some pointers:

1. Speak with a healthcare professional because It's crucial to speak with a healthcare professional before beginning any fasting routine, particularly if you're over 50, to make sure it's healthy for you and takes into account any potential medical issues or drugs you may be taking.

2. Increase the length of the fasting time gradually as your body becomes used to it. Start with shorter fasting intervals. By doing this, possible negative effects like weariness or irritation may be reduced.

3. Take into account time-restricted eating, as an alternative to more strenuous fasting regimens like extended or alternate-day fasting, take into account a time-restricted feeding strategy. For instance, restrict your

daily meals to an 8–10 hour window, such as 8 am–6 pm, and fast the rest of the time.

4. Put an emphasis on nutrient-dense meals in other to promote general health and supply vital vitamins and minerals, make sure to give nutrient-dense foods top priority throughout your eating window. Consume an abundance of fruits, veggies, whole grains, lean proteins, and healthy fats.

5. Remain hydrated and control hunger, drink lots of water during the fasting time.

6. Pay attention to your body: Observe how intermittent fasting affects your body. If you encounter any unfavorable side effects or if it doesn't seem right for you, think about changing your strategy or giving it up completely.

7. Be aware of hormonal changes, hormonal fluctuations, such as variations in estrogen levels during menopause, can affect women over 50. It's crucial to consider the potential effects of fasting on your body at this point in your life because these changes might have an influence on your hunger and metabolism.

8. Put your general health first keep in mind that intermittent fasting is only one facet of a healthy way of living. For general well-being, give top priority to obtaining enough sleep, controlling stress, engaging in physical activity, and preserving social relationships.

CHANGES IN HORMONES AND FASTING METHODS

The way the body reacts to fasting can be influenced by hormonal fluctuations, particularly in women. Women may customize their fasting techniques to meet their unique requirements and maximize the health advantages of fasting while maintaining hormonal balance and general well-being by being aware of how changes in hormones affect appetite and metabolism. In light of hormone fluctuations, you might think about the following fasting techniques:

MENOPAUSE:

Changes in hormones, such as a drop in oestrogen levels, can have an effect on body composition and metabolism. It's possible that during this period, women's reactions to fasting shift. Finding the most effective fasting strategy during menopause may include experimenting with various fasting protocols, such as shorter windows or less frequent fasting.

THYROID FUNCTION:

The metabolism is greatly influenced by thyroid hormones. To maintain thyroid health and general well-being, women with thyroid issues should work closely with a healthcare professional to monitor thyroid function and modify fasting techniques as needed

STRESS HORMONES

Prolonged stress can throw hormone balance out of whack, resulting in problems including dysregulated cortisol and heightened appetites. Fasting combined with stress-relieving techniques like yoga, meditation, or time spent in nature might help lessen the damaging effects of stress on hormonal health.

GROWTH HORMONE

Research has indicated that fasting raises growth hormone levels, which are important for metabolism, fat burning, and muscle maintenance. Periodic or intermittent fasting are two fasting techniques that may help certain women maximise their synthesis of growth hormones.

INSULIN SENSITIVITY

Women who have type 2 diabetes or insulin resistance may benefit most from fasting's ability to increase insulin sensitivity. To guarantee safe fasting practices, it is important to regularly monitor blood sugar levels and collaborate with a healthcare expert.

INDIVIDUAL VARIABILITY

Different people react differently to fasting on their hormones. It's critical to monitor your body's reaction and modify your fasting tactics as necessary. While some women may perform better with shorter or less frequent fasts, others may flourish with longer fasts.

<u>MEAL IDEAS AND RECIPES</u>

Here are some meal ideas and strategies to consider that are helpful tips for intermittent fasting and will also enable you to achieve a better result.

1. **Balanced meals:** Aim to include a balance of protein, healthy fats, fibre-rich carbohydrates, and vegetables in each meal to promote satiety and provide essential nutrients.

2. **Meal prep:** Spend some time each week planning and preparing meals in advance to make healthy eating more convenient. Cook larger batches of food that can be portioned out and stored for later use.

3. **Batch cooking:** Cook large quantities of grains, proteins, and vegetables that can be used as building blocks for multiple meals throughout the week. For example, roast a big batch of vegetables and use them in salads, stir-fries, or grain bowls.

4. **Portion control:** Pay attention to portion sizes to avoid overeating, especially when consuming calorie-dense foods. Use smaller plates and bowls to help control portion sizes and prevent mindless eating.

5. **Snack wisely:** Choose nutrient-dense snacks such as fruits, nuts, Greek yogurt, or vegetables with hummus to help curb hunger between meals and provide a steady source of energy.

6. **Include protein:** Protein-rich foods like lean meats, poultry, fish, tofu, beans, and lentils can help keep you feeling full and satisfied. Aim to include protein in each meal to support muscle maintenance and repair.

7. **Focus on whole foods:** Choose whole, minimally processed foods whenever possible, as they tend to be higher in nutrients and lower in added sugars, unhealthy fats, and sodium.

8. **Incorporate variety:** Experiment with different ingredients, flavors, and cuisines to keep meals interesting and prevent boredom. Try incorporating new fruits, vegetables, whole grains, and herbs and spices into your meals for added variety and flavor.

9.   **Mindful eating:** Practise mindful eating by slowing down, savoring each bite, and paying attention to hunger and fullness cues. This can help prevent overeating and promote a greater appreciation for food.

10.   **Stay hydrated:** Drink plenty of water throughout the day to stay hydrated and help prevent overeating, as thirst can sometimes be mistaken for hunger.

DELICIOUS RECIPES TAILORED FOR WOMEN OVER 50

In this session, I have skillfully selected recipes that will be very helpful for this course, delicious and filled with nutrients to support women in keeping fit. You can as well customize them base on personal preferences and dietary needs.

First on the list is SALMON AND QUINOA SALAD

SALMON AND QUINOA SALAD

Basic Ingredient

- One cup quinoa

- Two cups mixed salad greens - Two fish fillets

- Half a cup of cherry tomatoes - Diced cucumber

- One diced avocado

- 1/4 cup finely chopped red onion

- Two teaspoons of freshly chopped dill (or other preferred herb)

- One tablespoon of lemon juice

- Two teaspoons of olive oil

- To taste, add salt and pepper.

PROCEDURE

1.   Prepare the quinoa as directed on the box. After cooking, use a fork to fluff it up and allow it to cool to room temperature.

2.   Set the oven temperature to 375°F, or 190°C. Arrange the salmon fillets onto a parchment paper-lined baking sheet. Add a drizzle of olive oil and season with pepper and salt. Bake the salmon for 12 to 15 minutes, or until it is cooked through and flake readily when tested with a fork.

3.   As the salmon bakes, get the salad ingredients ready. Cooked quinoa, mixed salad greens, cherry tomatoes, cucumber, avocado, and red onion should all be combined in a big mixing dish.

4.   To create the dressing, combine the olive oil, lemon juice, chopped dill, salt, and pepper in a small dish.

5.   Take the salmon out of the oven and let it to cool a little. Next, break up the salmon into little pieces using a fork.

6.   Include the salmon flake in the salad mixture. To ensure that every item is uniformly coated, drizzle with the prepared dressing and gently toss.

7. Taste and, if necessary, adjust seasoning. If preferred, top the salmon and quinoa salad right away with more fresh herbs.

Savor your tasty and nourishing Quinoa and Salmon Salad!

VEGETABLE STIR-FRY WITH TOFU

This is a quick and delicious recipe for a stir-fried vegetable dish with tofu.

Basic Ingredients

- 400g of firm tofu, pressed and also drained
- One tablespoon of sesame oil
- Two tablespoons of vegetable oil – Soy sauce or tamari
- Three minced garlic cloves
- Grated fresh ginger, one tablespoon – Sliced bell pepper
- One carrot cut into matchstick shapes
- One cup of sliced mushrooms
- One cup of snap peas or snow peas
- 2 chopped green onions
- Prepared noodles or rice for serving.

REGARDING THE SAUCE

- One tablespoon of hoisin sauce
- Three teaspoons of soy sauce or tamari
- One tablespoon of rice vinegar
- One teaspoon of cornstarch
- One teaspoon of optional honey or maple syrup
- Two tsp of water

HOW TO PREPARE VEGETABLE STIR-FRY WITH TOFU

1. Begin by getting the tofu ready. Sliced tofu that has been compressed into cubes should be put on a shallow dish. Add a drizzle of 1 tablespoon sesame oil and 2 teaspoons soy sauce. Let the tofu lie in the marinade for ten to fifteen minutes after giving it a little toss to coat.

2. Combine all the sauce ingredients (soy sauce, hoisin sauce, rice vinegar, cornstarch, honey or maple syrup, if using), and water in a small dish. Put aside.

3. In a big skillet or wok, heat up one tablespoon of vegetable oil over medium-high heat. When brown and crispy, add the marinated tofu cubes and fry for 3–4 minutes on each side. After taking the tofu out of the skillet, set it aside.

4. Add the last tablespoon of vegetable oil to the same skillet. Add the grated ginger and minced garlic, and sauté until fragrant, approximately 1 minute.

5. Fill the skillet with the sliced bell pepper, snap peas, broccoli florets, and carrot matchsticks. Sauté the veggies for five to six minutes, or until they are soft yet still crunchy.

6. Place the cooked tofu back in the skillet with the veggies and cover with the prepared sauce. To uniformly coat everything with sauce, give it a good stir.

7. Simmer for a further two to three minutes, or until the sauce has slightly thickened and the food is well cooked.

8. Turn off the heat and top with finely chopped green onions.

9.   Top cooked rice or noodles with the hot vegetable stir-fry with tofu.

10.   Savor your tasty and nourishing stir-fried vegetables with tofu!

You are welcome to modify the veggies and sauce to suit your tastes. Have fun!

MEDITERRANEAN CHICKPEA SALAD

This is a light dish for chickpea salad from the Mediterranean:

Basic Ingredient

- Two cans of washed and drained chickpeas, 15 ounces each
- 1/2 red onion, coarsely chopped
- 1/2 cup chopped and pitted Kalamata olives
- 1 cup chopped cherry tomatoes
- 1/2 cup of crumbled feta cheese
- 1/4 cup of freshly chopped parsley
- 1/4 cup of optionally chopped mint
- One lemon's juice
- 2 minced garlic cloves
- 3 tablespoons extra virgin olive oil
- 1Salt and pepper to taste

HOW TO PREPARE MEDITERRANEAN CHICKPEA SALAD

1. Combine the chickpeas, diced cucumber, chopped red onion, split cherry tomatoes, sliced Kalamata olives, crumbled feta cheese, chopped parsley, and chopped mint (if using) in a large mixing bowl.

2. To create the dressing, combine the extra virgin olive oil, minced garlic, lemon juice, salt, and pepper in a small bowl.
3. Drizzle the chickpea salad with the dressing, tossing thoroughly to evenly cover all of the ingredients.
4. Add extra salt, pepper, or lemon juice to taste and adjust the seasoning if needed.
5. To let the flavors combine, let the salad sit at room temperature for 15 to 20 minutes.
6. You may serve the Mediterranean Chickpea Salad as a light supper or as a refreshing side dish. Have fun!

You can easily alter this salad by using other Mediterranean-inspired components like cubed avocado, artichoke hearts, or roasted red peppers. It's nourishing, adaptable, and a great choice for a healthy lunch or summertime get-together.

ROASTED VEGETABLE FRITTATA

Of course! This is a quick and easy recipe for a tasty frittata with roasted vegetables:

BASIC INGREDIENT

- One cup of mixed veggies, including mushrooms, onions, zucchini, and bell peppers
- Six big eggs

- 1/4 cup cream or milk
- Half a cup of shredded cheese, such mozzarella or cheddar

- Add salt and pepper.
- Use two teaspoons of olive oil.
- Optional fresh herb garnish, such as parsley or basil

HOW TO PREPARE ROASTED VEGETABLE FRITTATA

1. Set the oven temperature to 375°F, or 190°C.

2. Roughly chop the mixed veggies into bite-sized chunks.

3. Transfer the chopped veggies to a parchment paper-lined baking sheet. Add a drizzle of olive oil and season with pepper and salt. For an even coat, toss.

4. Roast the veggies for 20 to 25 minutes, or until they are soft and start to caramelize, in a preheated oven.

5. In a mixing dish, whisk together the eggs, grated cheese, and milk or cream while the veggies are roasting. Add pepper and salt for seasoning.
6. Take the veggies out of the oven once they have finished roasting and lower the oven's temperature to 350°F (175°C).

7. Turn up the heat to medium in an ovenproof skillet. Drizzle the skillet's bottom with a little olive oil.
8. Evenly distribute the roasted veggies in the pan after adding them.

9. Ensure that the veggies are equally spread by pouring the egg mixture over them in the skillet.
10. Simmer the frittata for three to four minutes, or until the sides begin to firm.

11. Place the pan in the oven that has been warmed, and bake for 12 to 15 minutes, or until the top of the frittata is golden brown and the middle is set.

12. After the frittata is done, take the pan out of the oven and let it to cool for a little while.

13. Cut the frittata into wedges, top with fresh herbs, if preferred, and serve warm or cold. Savor your tasty frittata with roasted vegetables!

GREEK YOGURT PARFAIT

Here's a quick and delectable Greek yogurt parfait recipe:

BASIC INGREDIENT

1. One cup of plain or flavored Greek yogurt, as desired
2. 1/2 cup granola (store-bought or homemade)
3. 1/2 cup of fresh blueberries, raspberries, and strawberries, among other mixed berries
4. One tablespoon (optional) of maple syrup or honey
5. One tablespoon of chopped nuts, optional (such as walnuts or almonds)

METHOD OF PREPARATION

1. Begin by arranging the ingredients in a dish or glass. Start at the bottom with a teaspoon of Greek yogurt.

2. Cover the yogurt with a coating of granola.

3. Add a layer of mixed berries after that.

4. Continue layering until you get to the top of the bowl or glass, then add one last layer of Greek yogurt.

5. If you'd like, drizzle some honey or maple syrup on top for more sweetness.

6. If preferred, garnish with chopped nuts for an added taste and crunch.

7. Present your mouth watering Greek yogurt parfait right now and savor it!

You may also add more toppings to your parfait, such shredded coconut, sliced bananas, or a dash of cinnamon. You may have this adaptable and healthful treat for breakfast, as a snack, or even as a light dessert.

CHAPTER FIVE

COMBINING INTERMITTENT FASTING WITH OTHER LIFESTYLE FACTORS

The total advantages and efficacy of intermittent fasting can be increased by combining it with other aspects of lifestyle. The following are some ways to combine intermittent fasting with other healthful lifestyle choices:

1. **Regular Exercise:** During your fast, make time for regular physical exercise. Enhancing metabolic health and optimizing fat burning are two benefits of fasting during exercise. For general fitness, aim for a mix of aerobic, strength, and flexibility workouts.

2. **Healthy meal:** To make sure your body is getting all the vital nutrients it needs, eat a balanced, nutrient-dense meal throughout the designated eating times. To support your health objectives, put an emphasis on nutritious foods including fruits, vegetables, whole grains, lean meats, and healthy fats.

3. **Hydration:** Make sure you stay well-hydrated by consuming lots of water throughout the day, particularly when you're fasting. For variation, you can also drink infused water, sparkling water, or herbal teas.

4. **Sufficient Sleep:** Make it a priority to have a sufficient amount of high-quality sleep every night, since it is essential for hormone control, metabolism, and general health. Set up a regular sleep pattern and try to get between seven and nine hours of sleep every night.

5. **Stress Management:** To assist lower stress levels, try stress-relieving activities like yoga, deep breathing exercises, meditation, or spending time in nature. Discovering efficient techniques to decompress and unwind is crucial as long-term stress can negatively affect hormone balance and metabolic health.

6. **Mindful Eating:** Utilize mindful eating techniques throughout mealtimes by being aware of your body's signals of hunger and fullness, enjoying every mouthful, and concentrating on the sensory aspects of eating. This can encourage a better connection with food and help avoid overindulging.

7. **Social Support:** During your fasting journey, surround yourself with encouraging friends, family, or members of online forums who have similar health objectives and can offer accountability and support.

8. **Frequent Health Examinations:** Make an appointment for routine checkups with your healthcare provider to keep an eye on your health, particularly if you take medication or have any underlying medical concerns. They may provide you individualized advice and assistance to make sure that fasting is suitable and safe for you.

<u>STRESS MANAGEMENT TECHNIQUES</u>

Incorporating these stress management tactics into your daily routine will help you better cope with stress and enhance your overall quality of life. Stress management is crucial for general well-being.

1. **Deep Breathing:** To trigger the body's relaxation response, engage in deep breathing exercises. Try taking four deep breaths through your nose, holding them for four counts, and then taking four calm breaths out through your mouth. Repeat many times.

2. **Mindfulness Meditation:** Practice mindfulness meditation to lower stress levels and develop present-moment awareness. Every day, set aside some time to sit still, concentrate on your breathing, and objectively watch your thoughts

3. **Progressive Muscle Relaxation:** To encourage both physical and mental relaxation, progressive muscle relaxation entails tensing and then releasing each muscle group in the body. Concentrate on one muscle group at a time, starting at your toes and working your way up to your head.

4. **Exercise:** Getting regular exercise helps elevate mood and lower stress levels. Include enjoyable exercises in your regular regimen, such as cycling, yoga, running, walking, or swimming.

5. **Healthy Lifestyle Practices:** Make it a priority to adopt healthy practices including cutting back on alcohol and caffeine, eating a balanced meal, getting enough sleep, and being hydrated. These routines promote resistance to stress and general well-being.

6. **Social Support:** During trying times, spend time with friends, relatives, or other encouraging people who can provide perspective, encouragement, and a listening ear. Making connections with other people can give one a sense of community and lessen feelings of loneliness.

7. **Time Management:** Make good use of time management strategies by prioritizing work, segmenting larger projects into smaller ones, and establishing reasonable objectives. To prevent feeling overburdened, refrain from taking on more than you can handle and have the ability to say no.

8. **Hobbies and Calm Activities:** Take up enjoyable and stress-relieving hobbies or pastimes, like cooking, reading, gardening, or spending time in nature. These pursuits can aid in detaching you from pressures and fostering a feeling of wellness

9. **Seeking expert Assistance:** If stress becomes too much for you to handle, think about getting help from a mental health expert, such a therapist or counselor. They may provide you support, coping mechanisms, and direction based on your unique requirements.

QUALITY SLEEP PRACTICES

A good night's sleep is crucial for general health and wellbeing. You may increase both the quantity and quality of your sleep, which will enhance your general health and wellbeing, by adopting these healthy sleeping habits into your daily routine.

1. **Create a Regular Sleep Schedule:** Even on weekends, go to bed and wake up at the same time every day. Maintaining consistency enhances the quality of your sleep by balancing your body's internal clock.

2. **Establish a Calm Bedtime habit:** Establish a peaceful nighttime habit to let your body know when it's time to unwind. This might involve doing things like reading, having a warm bath, using relaxation methods, or enjoying calming music.

3. **Establish a Comfortable Sleep Environment:** Keep your bedroom quiet, dark, and cold to ensure that it promotes restful sleep. To reduce distractions, choose a comfortable mattress and cushions and think about utilizing white noise generators or blackout curtains.

4. **Minimize Screen Time Before Bed:** At least one hour before going to bed, limit your time spent on electronic devices including computers, tablets, and cellphones. The hormone that controls sleep, melatonin, may be produced less effectively when blue light from screens is present.

5. **Pay Attention to Your Food and Drinks:** Avoid large meals, coffee, and alcohol just before bed because these might cause sleep disturbances. Choose herbal drinks and light nibbles instead. Additionally, drink plenty of water during the day, but cut back on liquids just before bed to avoid having to get up early to use the restroom.

6. **Exercise Frequently:** Get moving throughout the day, but steer clear of intense exercise just before bed because it might be stimulating. A little exercise in the morning might help you sleep better.

7. **Control Stress and Anxiety:** Before going to bed, try some relaxation techniques to assist you de-stress and clear your head, including progressive muscle relaxation, deep breathing, or meditation.

8. **Limit Naps:** Although quick naps can be helpful, particularly for senior citizens, avoid taking them in the late afternoon since this might disrupt your sleep at night.

9. **Allow Natural Light to Enter Your Body:** Throughout the day, especially in the morning, allow yourself to be exposed to natural sunshine. Better sleep-wake cycles are encouraged and your body's internal clock is regulated by natural light.

10. **Seek Professional Assistance if Needed:** If your sleep problems persist even after putting these strategies into practice, think about

consulting a medical professional or sleep expert who can assess underlying problems and offer suitable therapy.

<u>IMPORTANCE OF REGULAR PHYSICAL ACTIVITY</u>

At every stage of life, sustaining good health and well-being requires regular physical exercise. Including exercise in your daily routine may have a significant positive impact on your physical and emotional well-being, which can enhance your lifespan and quality of life.

1. **Enhances Physical Health:** Frequent exercise promotes cardiovascular health, increases endurance, and enhances general physical fitness by strengthening the heart, lungs, and muscles. Additionally, it lowers the chance of developing chronic illnesses including type 2 diabetes, heart disease, stroke, and several forms of cancer.

2. **Weight control:** By assisting in the burning of calories and maintenance of a healthy weight, physical exercise is essential for weight control. In addition, it can speed up metabolism and encourage fat loss—especially when paired with a healthy diet.

3. **Improves Mental Health:** Research has demonstrated that exercise improves mental health by lowering stress, anxiety, and depressive symptoms. It can also contribute to better general mental health by elevating mood, increasing self-esteem, and encouraging better sleep.

4. **Promotes Brain Health:** Research has shown a connection between regular exercise and enhanced cognitive performance as well as a lower chance of cognitive aging. Exercise helps lower the chance of acquiring neurodegenerative disorders like Alzheimer's disease and improve memory, concentration, and decision-making abilities.

5. **Boosts Energy Levels:** Regular exercise helps lower symptoms of exhaustion and boost energy levels. Increased vitality and endurance result from improved circulation and oxygen delivery to the muscles, tissues, and organs.

6. **Enhances Sleep Quality:** Physical activity can assist control sleep cycles and enhance the quality of sleep. Frequent exercise can improve

your ability to get asleep more quickly, remain asleep longer, and have deeper, more restorative sleep.

<u>CONCLUSION</u>

Finally, intermittent fasting offers women over 50 a viable way to improve their general health and wellbeing. Current research indicates possible advantages such enhanced metabolic health, weight control, and cognitive function, but further studies are needed to properly evaluate its long-term impacts and applicability for this population. Before starting an intermittent fasting regimen, women over 50 should speak with healthcare providers to be sure it is appropriate for their specific health issues and objectives. This is true of any dietary plan. In this group, intermittent fasting may be a useful strategy for fostering health and vitality if done with thoughtful thought and individualised direction.